SWEET DISRUPTION:

Unveiling Sugar's Impact on Men Beyond 36

.....Daniel's Journey

Dr. James Rim

Copyright © 2023 Dr.JamesRim

All rights reserved. No part of this publication, including the title "Sweet Disruption: Unveiling Sugar's Impact on Men Beyond 36", may be reproduced, distributed, or transmitted in any form or by any means, including photocopying, recording, or other electronic or mechanical methods, without the prior written permission of the publisher, except in the case of brief quotations embodied in critical reviews and certain other noncommercial uses permitted by copyright law.

Table of contents

Chapter 1

Introduction: Unveiling the Sweet Trap

Daniel sat at his kitchen table, staring at the plate of chocolate chip cookies in front of him. As he contemplated reaching for another cookie, a wave of unease washed over him. At 38, he found himself facing health concerns he had never imagined a few years ago. The reflection in the mirror didn't quite match the vibrant, energetic man he used to be.

His doctor's words echoed in his mind— elevated blood sugar levels, increasing cholesterol, and a stubborn waistline that seemed to expand no matter how much he exercised. "It's common at your age, "the doctor had said reassuringly, but there was something unsettling about being categorized as part of a demographic facing "common" health issues.

Turning away from the cookies, Daniel glanced at the family photo on the wall. His two young children reminded him of the active life he used to lead. Hiking trips, basketball games, and spontaneous adventures were now distant memories. The fast-paced demands of his career and the convenience of takeout had gradually eroded his once-healthy habits.

With a sigh, he leaned back in his chair, realizing that this phase of life demanded a fresh perspective. It wasn't just about shedding a few pounds or lowering his sugar intake—it was about reclaiming his vitality, about ensuring that the upcoming years would be as fulfilling as the ones that had come before.

As he thought about the future, a blend of determination and curiosity began to stir within Daniel. He reached for his smartphone and started typing, "Effects of sugar on men over 36" into the search bar. The journey to understand the complexities of sugar's impact had begun—a journey that would lead him to insights, challenges, and ultimately, a healthier path forward.

Health Landscape: The Changing Horizon of Midlife Wellness

In recent years, Daniel had noticed a shift in his priorities. The all-night parties of his twenties had given way to early mornings and responsible decisions. Alongside this natural progression came a newfound awareness of his health—a realization that his body, once so resilient, now seemed to demand more attention.

He wasn't alone in this journey. Across the globe, men over 36 were experiencing a similar evolution in their health concerns. It was a phase of life marked by subtle changes, both physical and metabolic, that often caught them off guard. The truth was, midlife health wasn't just about maintaining appearances—it was about safeguarding the body's internal mechanisms to ensure long-term vitality.

Cardiovascular Crossroads: Midlife often saw a rise in cardiovascular issues. Cholesterol levels that had been in check suddenly required monitoring, and the threat of heart disease loomed closer. The heart that had tirelessly powered them through life now demanded a recalibration of dietary choices and lifestyle.

Weight Woes: For many, the days of effortlessly maintaining a healthy weight seemed to slip away. It wasn't just about fitting into jeans—it was about the visceral fat that accumulated around the waistline, posing a risk to metabolic health. Midlife weight gain was more than just an aesthetic concern; it was a precursor to various health challenges.

Insidious Intolerance: As men aged, their relationship with certain foods altered. Foods that were once enjoyable, like rich desserts or indulgent treats, now had the potential to trigger digestive distress. Lactose intolerance, gluten sensitivity, and even mild allergies became more commonplace.

Energy Ebb and Flow: Energy levels took on a new rhythm. Instead of the boundless energy of youth, men over 36 found themselves experiencing fluctuations in vitality. Mornings might be invigorating, but afternoons brought an unexpected slump, making them question the demands of their daily routine.

Diabetes Dialogue: The "D" word—diabetes—was no longer a distant concern. Type 2 diabetes, once thought to affect only the elderly, was becoming increasingly prevalent in midlife. Blood sugar management demanded a new level of vigilance, making dietary choices a more critical consideration than ever before.

As men navigated this changing health landscape, one aspect became evident: the role of sugar was far more significant than they had initially assumed. Sugar, often dismissed as a mere indulgence, was emerging as a key player in the intricate interplay of midlife health challenges. What had seemed innocent in earlier years was revealing its potential to disrupt metabolic equilibrium and undermine wellness.

Chapter 2

The Sugar Maze: Navigating the Complexities of a Common Culprit

As Daniel delved into his quest to understand the impact of sugar on men over 36, he found himself navigating a labyrinth of information—a maze where the nuances of sugar's influence were as intricate as the human body itself. What had once seemed like a simple ingredient in his favorite treats now revealed itself as a complex culprit with far-reaching consequences.

Types of Sugars: The journey began with an exploration of the different types of sugars that populated his world. From the naturally occurring sugars in fruits to the refined sugars added to processed foods, Daniel learned that sugar wasn't a one-size-fits-all entity. Fructose, glucose, sucrose—the variations were numerous, each with its own metabolic implications.

Metabolic Dance: The metabolic dance between sugar and the body's intricate systems was one of the first revelations. As he delved into the science, Daniel discovered that the body responded differently to different types of sugars. The rapid spikes in blood sugar from sugary drinks triggered a cascade of events, leading to insulin release and potential energy crashes.

Insulin's Role: The spotlight shifted to insulin—the hormone that acted as a key player in the sugar metabolism process. Daniel learned about insulin's role in shuttling glucose into cells for energy, and the implications of insulin resistance. This newfound knowledge shed light on the connection between excessive sugar consumption and the development of conditions like type 2 diabetes.

Beyond Calories: Sugar's impact extended beyond its caloric content. Daniel was startled to learn that even "low-calorie" sugary snacks could disrupt his body's finely tuned balance. The intricacies of how sugar influenced hunger hormones and triggered cravings underscored that the story was more complex than simply counting calories.

Inflammation and Beyond: One of the most profound revelations was sugar's role in inflammation—a process that had implications for a range of health concerns, from cardiovascular disease to joint pain. Daniel realized that the seemingly innocent indulgences were contributing to a state of chronic inflammation that could set the stage for long-term health challenges.

Mindful Consumption: Armed with a deeper understanding of the sugar maze, Daniel saw the importance of mindful consumption. It wasn't about demonizing sugar outright, but about recognizing its impact and making choices that aligned with his health goals. He found himself empowered to decode food labels, identify hidden sugars, and make informed decisions about what he put into his body.

Navigating the sugar maze had been a journey of revelations and insights for Daniel. What had once been a simple indulgence now stood as a powerful player in his health equation. The intricate web of sugar's influence had been unveiled, and armed with knowledge,

Daniel was ready to tread more consciously along his path to health and well-being.

Chapter 3

Midlife Metabolism: Sugar's Unique Impact

As Daniel journeyed deeper into his exploration of sugar's effects, he encountered a pivotal realization—the intricate relationship between his midlife metabolism and the way his body processed sugar. No longer could he rely on the metabolism of his youth; midlife brought about changes that demanded a nuanced understanding of sugar's impact.

The Changing Landscape: Daniel learned that metabolism was far from a static process—it evolved with age. His once-speedy metabolism that effortlessly burned off calories was giving way to a more deliberate pace. This shift was accompanied by a decrease in muscle mass and a tendency for excess calories to be stored as fat—changes that had profound implications for how his body handled sugar.

Insulin Resistance Emerges: The concept of insulin resistance emerged as a focal point in understanding sugar's unique impact. As Daniel approached midlife, his cells were becoming less responsive to the hormone insulin, which played a central role in sugar regulation. The result? Higher blood sugar levels after meals, leading to energy crashes and potential long-term health issues.

Weight Woes and Waistlines: Daniel recognized that midlife weight gain wasn't just an aesthetic concern—it was deeply connected to his metabolism and sugar metabolism. The accumulation of visceral fat around his waistline was a hallmark of this phase, and it had the potential to exacerbate insulin resistance, forming a vicious cycle that demanded his attention.

Energy Levels and Mood Swings: The intricate dance between metabolism and sugar extended to his energy levels and mood. The dips and spikes he experienced throughout the day were intricately linked to his body's ability to regulate sugar. Understanding this connection shed light on the afternoon slumps and mood swings he often grappled with.

Nutrient Needs and Sugar Choices: Midlife metabolism brought with it altered nutrient needs. Daniel realized that his body's demand for certain vitamins and minerals, like magnesium and chromium, became more pronounced as he aged. These nutrients played essential roles in sugar metabolism, prompting him to make more conscious choices about his diet to support his changing needs.

Strategies for Balance: Armed with the knowledge of his evolving metabolism, Daniel embarked on a journey to balance his sugar intake. He discovered the power of fiber-rich foods and complex carbohydrates in moderating blood sugar spikes. He also recognized the importance of regular physical activity in enhancing insulin sensitivity and metabolism.

Through his exploration of midlife metabolism and sugar's unique impact, Daniel uncovered the intricate ways in which his body's response to sugar had evolved. The awareness that his choices weren't just about indulgence but were intertwined with his metabolic health gave him the tools to navigate his sugar consumption with greater precision, setting the stage for a healthier and more balanced future.

Chapter 4

Beyond the Sweet Tooth: Emotional and Psychological Aspects

As Daniel's journey into the world of sugar unfolded, he found himself peeling back layers that extended far beyond mere taste. The allure of sugary treats wasn't solely about flavor—it was a doorway into a realm of emotions, memories, and intricate psychological connections that he had never fully considered.

Comfort in Every Bite: Daniel discovered that sugary indulgences often provided more than just a sensory experience; they offered comfort in times of stress, loneliness, or even celebration. The warmth of nostalgia associated with a childhood dessert or the temporary respite from life's challenges—sugar became a source of emotional solace.

Emotions and Cravings: As he delved deeper, Daniel recognized the undeniable link between emotions and cravings. Stress and anxiety could trigger an intense desire for sweets, offering a brief escape from emotional turmoil. The act of consuming sugar had become intertwined with the emotional states he encountered daily.

The Dopamine Rush: One of the most intriguing revelations was the connection between sugar and dopamine, the brain's "feel-good" neurotransmitter. Indulging in sugary foods triggered a surge of dopamine, creating a momentary rush of pleasure. This physiological response explained the allure of sugary treats as a means to experience moments of happiness.

Escaping the Cycle: Unveiling the emotional and psychological layers of sugar led Daniel to recognize a cycle—a pattern where consuming sugar temporarily elevated mood, only to be followed by a subsequent crash. This crash often triggered renewed cravings for sugar, perpetuating a cycle that left him seeking relief from both emotional and physical discomfort.

Mindful Consumption: Armed with this newfound awareness, Daniel began to embrace mindful consumption. He learned to differentiate between true hunger and emotional triggers, to recognize when he was seeking solace in sugar, and to find healthier ways to address his emotional needs. The practice of mindfulness extended beyond what he ate—it encompassed why he ate.

Empowerment Through Understanding: The exploration of sugar's emotional and psychological dimensions was a journey of empowerment. Daniel realized that he held the power to break free from the cycle of emotional eating, to choose alternatives that supported his well-being, and to cultivate a more balanced relationship with sugary foods.

As he journeyed through the emotional and psychological aspects of sugar consumption, Daniel wasn't merely confronting his sweet tooth—he was delving into the depths of his own emotional landscape. Through self-awareness, mindfulness, and a deeper understanding of the connections between sugar and his emotions, he was crafting a healthier and more harmonious way of nourishing both his body and his mind.

Chapter 5

Hidden Sugars: Unmasking Unseen Threats

As Daniel delved deeper into his quest to understand the impact of sugar on his health, he found himself on a journey of revelation—one that exposed the hidden sugars lurking in his daily diet. What had initially seemed innocent and harmless turned out to be an intricate web of unseen threats, challenging his perception of sugar consumption.

Beyond the Obvious: The realization that sugar was more than just the spoonful he added to his coffee was a sobering one. Daniel learned that hidden sugars—those stealthily tucked away in seemingly innocent foods— were pervasive and impactful. The fruit-flavored yogurt he enjoyed, the store-bought salad dressing he drizzled, and even the granola bars he considered a healthy snack—all contained hidden sugars that added up over time.

Disguised Delights: Delving into food labels, Daniel began to decipher the various aliases that sugar adopted to hide its presence. Words like "sucrose," "fructose," and "corn syrup" seemed innocuous, but they were all indicators of added sugars. Even seemingly health-conscious options were not immune—organic fruit juices, energy drinks, and whole-grain cereals often harbored hidden sugars that went unnoticed.

The Dangers of Overconsumption: Daniel discovered that hidden sugars weren't merely a dietary inconvenience—they posed real health risks. The cumulative effect of consuming these sugars could lead to weight gain, blood sugar spikes, and an increased risk of chronic conditions like type 2 diabetes and heart disease. What had once seemed like small indulgences now held the potential for long-term consequences.

Mindful Label Reading: Armed with this knowledge, Daniel adopted a new habit—meticulously reading food labels. He scrutinized the ingredient lists, seeking out hidden sugars and making more informed choices. The revelation that he had the power to control his sugar intake through awareness and label literacy was both empowering and eye-opening.

Alternatives and Strategies: Daniel's journey of uncovering hidden sugars led him to explore alternatives. He discovered that he could make his own salad dressing using simple ingredients, opt for whole fruits instead of fruit juices, and create satisfying snacks using nuts and seeds. These alternatives not only reduced his hidden sugar intake but also introduced him to the joys of preparing fresh and wholesome foods.

Empowerment Through Awareness: The exploration of hidden sugars was more than a lesson in label reading—it was a journey of empowerment. Armed with the ability to unmask unseen threats, Daniel was equipped to make choices that aligned with his health goals. By shedding light on the covert presence of hidden sugars, he was taking charge of his dietary decisions and shaping a healthier path forward.

Chapter 6

Health Impacts: From Heart to Hormones

As Daniel delved deeper into his investigation of sugar's influence, he uncovered a sprawling web of health impacts that extended far beyond his initial expectations. What had begun as a simple exploration into sugar's effects evolved into a comprehensive understanding of how sugar reached into nearly every facet of his well-being.

Cardiovascular Conundrums: At the forefront of the health impacts lay the intricate relationship between sugar and cardiovascular health. Daniel discovered that excessive sugar consumption wasn't just about empty calories—it was a significant contributor to heart disease. The inflammation triggered by sugar could damage blood vessels, increase cholesterol levels, and set the stage for arterial plaque buildup.

Weight Woes and Metabolic Mayhem: The journey further revealed the intricate dance between sugar and weight management. The role of insulin, the hormone responsible for regulating blood sugar, became central. Excessive sugar intake could lead to insulin resistance—a condition that impeded weight loss efforts and increased the risk of obesity.

Energy Ebb and Flow: Daniel came to understand the peaks and troughs of energy that punctuated his days weren't solely due to lack of sleep or workload. Sugar played a role in these energy fluctuations. Rapid spikes in blood sugar from sugary foods led to corresponding energy crashes, leaving him feeling tired and drained.

Hormonal Havoc: The exploration of sugar's impact on health unveiled its role in hormonal harmony—or lack thereof. The hormone insulin, intimately connected to sugar regulation, could influence other hormones like cortisol and estrogen. Disruptions in these hormonal interactions had implications for stress management, mood stability, and even reproductive health.

Gut Matters: Daniel was surprised to find that even his gut health was intertwined with sugar consumption. Excessive sugar intake could alter the balance of gut bacteria, leading to an imbalance in the gut microbiome. This disruption had far-reaching implications, from digestion issues to weakened immunity.

The Power of Moderation: As he unraveled the interconnected web of health impacts, Daniel realized that the message wasn't about complete sugar elimination—it was about moderation and informed choices. The empowerment lay in recognizing the consequences of his dietary decisions and navigating a path that balanced enjoyment with mindful consumption.

Armed with this comprehensive understanding of the health impacts of sugar, Daniel was making choices that reached beyond taste preferences. The journey had transformed his perspective on food, illuminating the hidden complexities that sugar brought to his physical, emotional, and hormonal well-being. By embracing this holistic perspective, he was setting the stage for a more conscious and health-centric future.

Chapter 7

Balancing Act: Crafting a Sugar-Conscious Diet

As Daniel's journey through the realm of sugar continued, he recognized that the path to better health was a delicate balancing act—a mindful interplay between enjoyment and well-being. The concept of a sugar-conscious diet emerged as a pivotal strategy, guiding him toward a harmonious relationship with sugar that prioritized both his taste preferences and his long-term wellness.

Quality Over Quantity: Daniel realized that the focus wasn't solely on reducing the quantity of sugar consumed, but on the quality of the sugars he chose. He learned to distinguish between naturally occurring sugars found in whole fruits and the added sugars prevalent in processed foods. This shift in perspective enabled him to make informed choices about where his sugar intake came from.

Whole-Food Focus: The heart of a sugar-conscious diet lay in embracing whole, unprocessed foods. Daniel discovered that these foods offered a wealth of nutrients, fiber, and natural sweetness that contributed to satiety and stable blood sugar levels. Filling his plate with colorful vegetables, whole grains, lean proteins, and healthy fats became a cornerstone of his approach.

Decoding Labels: Navigating the supermarket aisle became an exercise in label decoding. Armed with knowledge about the hidden names for sugar, Daniel learned to identify products with minimal added sugars. He found satisfaction in selecting foods with recognizable ingredients and steering clear of heavily processed options.

Mindful Indulgence: Balancing a sugar-conscious diet didn't mean completely forgoing indulgences. Daniel discovered the art of mindful indulgence—savoring a small piece of chocolate or enjoying a homemade dessert in moderation. This approach allowed him to enjoy the pleasures of sweetness while remaining aligned with his health goals.

Preparation Power: Meal planning and preparation became his allies in the sugar-conscious journey. By preparing his meals at home, Daniel had control over the ingredients he used and the sugar content of his dishes. He found joy in experimenting with herbs, spices, and natural sweeteners to enhance flavor without relying on excessive sugar.

Community and Connection: Daniel recognized that his sugar-conscious journey wasn't solitary. Engaging with a community of like-minded individuals provided support, recipe ideas, and a sense of camaraderie. Sharing successes and challenges in navigating a sugar-conscious diet strengthened his commitment to the lifestyle.

A Sustainable Lifestyle: The ultimate revelation was that a sugar-conscious diet wasn't a fleeting fad—it was a sustainable lifestyle choice that resonated with his well-being. Through mindful choices, education, and a deeper understanding of his body's response to sugar, Daniel was crafting a dietary approach that supported his long-term health and vitality.

Chapter 8

Sweet Solutions: Practical Tips for Cutting Back

As Daniel embarked on his journey to reduce sugar intake, he realized that the process required more than just willpower—it demanded practical strategies and actionable steps. The pursuit of a healthier relationship with sugar led him to discover a toolkit of sweet solutions designed to make the transition smoother and more sustainable.

1. Gradual Reduction: Daniel understood that abrupt changes could be overwhelming. Instead, he opted for a gradual approach, steadily decreasing sugar intake over time. This allowed his taste buds to adjust and reduced the likelihood of feeling deprived.

2. Read Labels: The habit of reading food labels became a powerful tool. Daniel scrutinized ingredient lists, looking for added sugars under various names. Armed with label literacy, he made conscious choices and was less likely to be caught off guard by hidden sugars.

3. Choose Whole Foods: Embracing whole, unprocessed foods played a central role. Fruits, vegetables, lean proteins, and whole grains became the foundation of his meals. These nutrient-rich choices not only satisfied his hunger but also minimized the need for added sugars.

4. Natural Sweeteners: Exploring natural sweeteners like honey, maple syrup, and stevia allowed Daniel to enjoy sweetness without the excessive sugar content. These alternatives provided a touch of sweetness while offering additional nutrients and flavors.

5. Mindful Snacking: Snacking mindfully helped Daniel avoid impulsive sugar-laden choices. He kept nutritious options, such as nuts, seeds, and cut-up vegetables, readily available. This way, he could satiate his hunger without resorting to sugary snacks.

6. Portion Control: Daniel learned that portion control was key to enjoying treats without overindulging. By savoring smaller portions of sugary foods, he could satisfy his cravings without experiencing energy crashes or excessive sugar intake.

7. Hydration: Staying hydrated played a surprising role in managing sugar cravings. Drinking plenty of water helped curb hunger and reduced the tendency to reach for sugary snacks out of boredom or thirst.

8. Mindful Eating: Slowing down and savoring each bite allowed Daniel to become more attuned to his body's signals. He learned to differentiate between true hunger and emotional triggers, enabling him to make conscious choices about when and what to eat.

9. Food Substitutions: Daniel found joy in exploring food substitutions. He replaced sugary beverages with herbal teas, swapped sugary cereals for whole-grain options, and experimented with recipes that used alternative flours and sweeteners.

10. Celebrate Progress: Celebrating milestones and successes was an important aspect of Daniel's journey. Each step he took toward reducing sugar intake was a victory. Recognizing and celebrating these achievements reinforced his commitment to his health goals.

Through these practical sweet solutions, Daniel found himself equipped with the tools needed to make lasting changes in his relationship with sugar. The journey was no longer about deprivation; it was about empowerment and a newfound sense of control over his dietary choices. With each sweet solution he embraced, Daniel was crafting a healthier and more balanced way of nourishing his body and mind.

Chapter 9

Empowering Change: Lifestyle Shifts for Lasting Impact

As Daniel's journey through sugar's complexities continued, he realized that the transformation he sought extended beyond dietary adjustments—it encompassed broader lifestyle shifts that would have a lasting impact on his well-being. These lifestyle shifts were about embracing a holistic approach that addressed not only what he ate but also how he lived.

1. Active Living: Daniel understood that a sedentary lifestyle could exacerbate the effects of sugar consumption. Regular physical activity became a cornerstone of his journey. Whether it was brisk walks, yoga sessions, or engaging in his favorite sports, exercise became a joyful way to support his health and metabolism.

2. Stress Management: The connection between stress and sugar cravings was undeniable. Daniel adopted stress management techniques such as deep breathing, meditation, and mindfulness. By taming stress, he minimized the emotional triggers that led to sugary indulgences.

3. Quality Sleep: Prioritizing quality sleep became a non-negotiable. Daniel recognized that insufficient sleep disrupted hormonal balance, increased cravings, and impaired metabolism. Creating a sleep-conducive environment and adhering to a consistent sleep schedule had profound effects on his well-being.

4. Mind-Body Connection: Daniel explored the mind-body connection, recognizing that his emotional state influenced his dietary choices. Practices like meditation and journaling helped him foster self-awareness, allowing him to address emotional triggers and make conscious decisions about sugar consumption.

5. Social Support: Engaging with a supportive community was vital. Daniel found that sharing his journey with friends, family, or online groups provided encouragement, recipe ideas, and a sense of accountability. The collective wisdom and shared experiences reinforced his commitment.

6. Learning and Growth: Education remained a powerful tool. Daniel continued to expand his knowledge about sugar's impact, delving into scientific research and seeking expert advice. This continuous learning empowered him to make informed decisions and advocate for his own health.

7. Mindful Eating Habits: Beyond what he ate, how he ate mattered. Daniel practiced mindful eating—savoring each bite, chewing slowly, and paying attention to hunger and fullness cues. This approach not only enhanced his enjoyment of meals but also fostered a deeper connection with his body's needs.

8. Prioritizing Self-Care: Daniel embraced self-care as a non-negotiable aspect of his journey. Whether it was reading, spending time in nature, or engaging in creative pursuits, he recognized that nurturing his well-being was essential for maintaining a balanced lifestyle.

9. Setting Realistic Goals: Instead of aiming for perfection, Daniel focused on setting realistic and achievable goals. This prevented feelings of failure and frustration, allowing him to celebrate small victories and maintain a positive outlook.

10. Celebrating Progress: Each step forward was a reason to celebrate. Whether it was a week of reduced sugar intake, an improved mood, or increased energy levels, Daniel acknowledged and celebrated his progress. This positive reinforcement fueled his motivation and commitment.

Through these lifestyle shifts, Daniel was transforming his relationship with sugar from one of indulgence to one of conscious choice. He understood that the path to lasting impact required a comprehensive approach—one that addressed his physical, emotional, and mental well-being. By embracing these lifestyle shifts, Daniel was not only shaping his present but also laying the foundation for a healthier and more empowered future.

Chapter 10

Nurturing Longevity: Exploring Sugar's Role in Aging Gracefully

As Daniel delved into the intricacies of sugar's impact, he uncovered a profound connection between his dietary choices and the way he aged. The concept of aging gracefully took on new dimensions as he realized that his relationship with sugar played a pivotal role in nurturing longevity and ensuring his well-being well into the future.

1. **Skin and Collagen**: The impact of sugar on collagen—the protein responsible for skin elasticity—captured Daniel's attention. He learned that excess sugar consumption could lead to a process called glycation, which damaged collagen and accelerated skin aging.

By moderating his sugar intake, he was safeguarding his skin's youthful appearance.

2. Cellular Aging: The exploration of cellular aging shed light on how sugar influenced the process. Excessive sugar intake could promote oxidative stress and inflammation, accelerating cellular damage and leading to premature aging. By reducing sugar consumption, Daniel was potentially slowing down the rate at which his cells aged.

3. Cognitive Health: The connection between sugar and cognitive health was eye-opening. Research suggested that diets high in sugar could increase the risk of cognitive decline and conditions like Alzheimer's disease. With this knowledge, Daniel saw the importance of nurturing his brain health through mindful sugar consumption.

4. Energy Levels: As he aged, Daniel recognized that stable energy levels were crucial for maintaining an active lifestyle. The fluctuations caused by sugar crashes could disrupt his ability to engage in physical activity and fully enjoy life. By managing his sugar intake, he was investing in sustained vitality.

5. Bone Health: Sugar's impact on bone health surprised him. Excessive sugar intake could lead to calcium depletion and weakened bones, contributing to osteoporosis. Recognizing the importance of strong bones for longevity, Daniel became more intentional about his sugar choices.

6. Inflammation and Chronic Disease: Understanding the role of sugar in inflammation offered a broader perspective on aging gracefully. Chronic inflammation was linked to a range of age-related diseases, from heart disease to arthritis. By mitigating inflammation through mindful sugar consumption, Daniel was taking a proactive step toward longevity.

7. Long-Term Independence: One of the most profound revelations was the impact of sugar on overall vitality and independence in old age. By making conscious choices about sugar consumption, Daniel was safeguarding his ability to enjoy an active and independent life well into his later years.

8. Embracing Nutrient-Rich Foods: With a focus on longevity, Daniel embraced nutrient-rich foods that supported his health. He filled his plate with antioxidants, vitamins, and minerals from colorful fruits and vegetables, lean proteins, and whole grains.

This approach nourished his body and provided the building blocks for healthy aging.

9. Cultivating a Positive Mindset: The journey of aging gracefully wasn't solely about physical health—it also encompassed a positive mindset. Daniel understood that his relationship with food and sugar played a role in fostering a healthy perspective on aging. By making choices aligned with his well-being, he was nurturing his self-esteem and confidence.

Through this exploration of sugar's role in aging gracefully, Daniel was crafting a blueprint for a vibrant and fulfilling life as he grew older. The knowledge that his choices today could influence his well-being in the years to come empowered him to make intentional decisions about his sugar consumption. By embracing this holistic approach, Daniel was nurturing his longevity and setting the stage for a future of health, vitality, and graceful aging.

Chapter 11

Community and Support: Building a Sugar-Awake Network for Success

Daniel's journey into a sugar-conscious lifestyle was enriched by the realization that he didn't have to navigate it alone. The power of community and support became evident as he embarked on the path of mindful sugar consumption. Building a sugar-awake network provided him with encouragement, accountability, and a shared sense of purpose.

1. Shared Experiences: Connecting with like-minded individuals who were also on their sugar-conscious journeys allowed Daniel to share his triumphs and challenges. Hearing stories from others who faced similar struggles fostered a sense of camaraderie and reassured him that he wasn't alone in his efforts.

2. Recipe Exchange: Within the sugar-awake community, Daniel found a treasure trove of recipe ideas that were both delicious and health-conscious. From inventive breakfast options to guilt-free desserts, the collective wisdom of the community expanded his culinary horizons and made his sugar-conscious lifestyle more enjoyable.

3. Accountability Partners: Having an accountability partner or group provided an extra layer of motivation. Daniel found that sharing his goals and progress with someone else encouraged him to stay on track. Whether it was a friend, family member, or online group, the support he received kept him committed.

4. Emotional Support: The journey to reducing sugar intake wasn't always smooth sailing. There were moments of temptation, frustration, and self-doubt. The sugar-awake network offered Daniel a safe space to express his emotions, seek advice, and receive encouragement from those who understood his struggles.

5. Problem-Solving Together: When faced with challenges or dilemmas, the sugar-awake community became a valuable resource. Daniel could seek guidance on deciphering food labels, managing cravings, and navigating social situations where sugary treats were abundant. The collective knowledge of the group was empowering.

6. Celebrating Milestones: Every victory, no matter how small, was a reason to celebrate within the sugar-awake network.

From reducing sugar intake for a week to successfully navigating a special event without overindulging, the community celebrated these achievements and provided positive reinforcement.

7. Motivation and Inspiration:
Interacting with others who were committed to a sugar-conscious lifestyle inspired Daniel to stay dedicated. Seeing the progress and success of fellow community members fueled his motivation and reminded him of the rewards that came from making mindful choices.

8. Lifelong Friendships: Beyond the shared goal of reducing sugar intake, Daniel formed meaningful connections with individuals who became friends for life. The bonds forged within the sugar-awake community extended beyond dietary choices, creating a sense of belonging and connection.

9. Paying It Forward: As Daniel experienced the benefits of community and support, he realized the importance of paying it forward. He became an active participant in the sugar-awake network, offering advice, sharing his journey, and providing encouragement to newcomers.

Through the power of community and support, Daniel's sugar-conscious journey transformed from a solitary effort into a shared endeavor. The sugar-awake network became a source of strength, inspiration, and connection that enriched his pursuit of a healthier relationship with sugar. By fostering these connections, Daniel not only empowered himself but also contributed to the collective well-being of the sugar-awake community.

Chapter 12

Conclusion: A Sweet Future - Navigating the Journey Ahead

As Daniel's journey through the intricate landscape of sugar came to a close, he found himself standing at the threshold of a new beginning—a future shaped by the insights, choices, and transformations he had experienced. The conclusion of this chapter marked not just an end, but the dawn of a sweet future, guided by wisdom and empowerment.

Reflection and Growth: Looking back on his voyage, Daniel recognized the immense growth he had undergone. From understanding the nuances of sugar's impact to making practical shifts in his lifestyle, he had evolved into a more conscious and empowered individual. The journey had been one of reflection, adaptation, and a continuous thirst for knowledge.

A Balanced Relationship: The conclusion wasn't about complete sugar elimination, but about achieving a balanced relationship with sugar. Daniel had learned that sugar could be enjoyed in moderation and that mindful choices were the cornerstone of a healthy approach. By understanding his body's needs and his personal triggers, he was able to make decisions aligned with his well-being.

Empowerment and Agency: One of the most profound takeaways from the journey was the sense of empowerment Daniel felt. Armed with knowledge, practical strategies, and a supportive community, he had reclaimed agency over his dietary decisions.

The choices he made were no longer influenced solely by habit or societal norms—they were deliberate and informed choices that supported his health.

A Blueprint for Others: As Daniel embraced this sweet future, he recognized that his journey was a blueprint for others seeking a more mindful and health-conscious approach to sugar. His exploration of sugar's impact, the strategies he employed, and the wisdom he gained could serve as a guide for those embarking on a similar path.

A Lifelong Commitment: The conclusion marked not the end of a chapter, but the beginning of a lifelong commitment. Daniel understood that the journey to mindful sugar consumption was ongoing—a journey that would evolve as he grew, learned, and adapted. The lessons he had learned would continue to shape his choices and contribute to his well-being.

Gratitude and Optimism: The conclusion was infused with gratitude for the journey itself. Daniel was thankful for the challenges, revelations, and moments of triumph that had accompanied him. As he looked ahead, he did so with optimism—knowing that the sweet future he was crafting was a reflection of his dedication to his health and a testament to his capacity for positive change.

In closing this chapter, Daniel embarked on the next phase of his journey with a heart full of gratitude and a spirit of anticipation. The lessons he had learned about sugar's impact and his own resilience would remain as guiding lights, illuminating the path to a future characterized by vitality, empowerment, and a harmonious relationship with food.